Super Backache Cure

Table of Contents

INTRODUCTION 3

CHAPTER 1: WHAT IS BACK PAIN AND WHY DOES IT OCCUR? 6

CHAPTER 2: SIMPLE EXERCISES TO PREVENT THE CAUSES OF BACK PAIN 13

CHAPTER 3: HOW TO IMPROVE YOUR POSTURE TO AVOID BACK PAIN 20

CHAPTER 4: THE BASIC YOGA POSES FOR RELIEVING BACK PAIN NATURALLY 27

CHAPTER 5: ALTERNATIVE TREATMENTS FOR LONG-TERM RELIEF FROM BACK PAIN 34

CONCLUSION 39

Introduction

I want to thank you and congratulate you for downloading the book, "Super Backache Cure: Chronic Back Pain Relief and Healing, Low Back Pain Fix, Self-Treatment and Care, Specific Exercises for Backache and Massage to Feel Better".

This book contains proven steps and strategies on how to relieve back pain by making suitable changes to your posture and with the help of some exercises.

We will also discuss some yoga asanas and alternative treatments for relieving back pain naturally.

Thanks again for downloading this book, I hope you enjoy it!

Chapter 1: What is back pain and why does it occur?

If there is one factor that can affect your life severely, even when subtle, then it is back pain. Whether mild, moderate or severe, backache can prevent you from carrying out your routine activity and even won't allow you to enjoy your life to the fullest.

And in case, the back pain becomes worse, your life could take a worse turn by limiting your movements and increasing your risk of complications.

Back pain is also one of the common reasons for the absence from work and seeking medical intervention. It can be highly uncomfortable as well as debilitating.

Back pain can affect the people of any age, and for different reasons. The risk of developing lower back pain can increase with advancing age. This age-related risk factor is often contributed by your previous occupation and the degenerative changes in your back that weaken the intervertebral disk between the vertebral bone in your back.

The lower back pain is also linked to the abnormalities of the lumbar spine, ligaments located around the spine and the discs, nerves, spinal cord, the muscles in this region, lower back muscles, pelvic and abdominal organs, and also the skin around your lumbar area.

In short, it is not just the bones that cause back pain, but even the organs in your body, the skin, and other tissues!

Hence, it is very important to never ignore back pain, and take steps to relieve it.

In this book, we will learn some simple exercises and natural remedies to relieve back pain. However, before this, it is important to know why back pain occurs in the first place.

Here is a glimpse of various causes of back pain most of which could be related to your faulty lifestyle.

What are the causes of back pain?

Strain

This is the most common cause of acute or short-lasting back pain. It usually stems from a sudden or excessive strain on your back that results in tension, and injury. The common causes of back pain related to strain include:

- Injuries, fractures, and falls

- Strained ligaments and muscles

- An increased muscle tension

- Muscle spasms

- Damaged intervertebral disks

Some of the activities that may be responsible for causing strains and spasms in your back include:

- Making an abrupt and awkward movement

- Lifting something that is too heavy

- Lifting something improperly

Structural problems

Structural problems in the back can also be the cause of excessive strain on the back muscles and bones resulting in back pain.
Some of these include:

- Ruptured disks: All the vertebrae in your spine are cushioned by disks to protect them against shocks and jerks. The rupture of these disks can deprive your back of the protective mechanisms resulting in more pressure on the muscles and nerves resulting in back pain.

- Bulging disks: When the discs bulge backward, they exert pressure on the nerves that pass through the spaces between 2 vertebrae. This can result in more pressure on the nerves and cause pain in the back and legs.

- Sciatica: Sciatica refers to a sharp, shooting pain that radiates to the lower back through the buttock along the back of the leg. The pain may run till the ankles or heels and cause severe discomfort and irritation. This cause of back pain is related to the herniated or bulging disc pressing on the sciatic nerve.

- Arthritis: Osteoarthritis is a major cause of back pain in obese individuals. It occurs due to the inflammation at the ends of the bones that becomes worse when they rub against each other during movements.

  It usually affects the thighs and knees as these are the weight-bearing bones of your body and hence, are likely to suffer damage due to the entire body weight exerted on them.

  If not managed properly, osteoarthritis can worsen over a period of time resulting in severe loss of mobility. When Osteoarthritis affects the bones in the back, the space around the spinal cord is narrowed due to the inflammatory changes like swelling. This condition is called spinal stenosis.

- Abnormal curvatures of the spine: the spinal column of a human body is designed to have a unique curvature to help us maintain balance and prevent falling. An abnormal curvature of the spine can increase the risk of back pain as it produces more strain on your muscles to maintain balance.

Besides these, there are a few factors that can cause or worsen back pain. These factors are related to your lifestyle, and hence easily modifiable. Let us learn more about such causes of back pain that you can easily avoid by making healthy changes to your lifestyle.

Modifiable causes of back pain

Your movements and posture

The most common modifiable cause of back pain results from your everyday activities and poor posture. These activities produce more strain on the muscles in the back and cause backache.
Some of the examples include:

- Sitting in a hunched position while working on computers

- Severe coughing and sneezing

- Over-stretching to reach out to something

- Bending forward, backward and sideward awkwardly

- Bending for long periods

- Lifting, pushing, pulling, and carrying a heavy load

- Sitting or standing for long periods

- Straining your neck forward, while driving

- Sleeping on a mattress which does not support your body or keep your spine straight

Living a tech-dependent life

You are more likely to suffer from back pain if you are a screen-king. Whether it is your television, laptop, or smartphones, the longer time you spent with these gadgets, the higher would be your risk of developing back pain.

Sleeping on your stomach

Sleeping on the sides or back can keep your spine neutral and elongated. But, if you have a habit of snoozing on your tummy, the strain on your back muscles increases making you prone to backache.

Ignoring the core

Your core is composed of much more than just the 6-pack abs. It also includes the muscles in your back, and sides. These muscles, along with your abs, allow you to stand upright, twist, bend, and rotate.

If you work out only your abs, and ignore the other muscles in your core, they will stay weak and less developed causing back pain.

Choosing inappropriate footwear

Sky-high stilettos are surely a no-no if you want to protect your back. However, it turns out that even flats can cause trouble. And flip-flops and sandals do provide a little arch support.
Hence, you are advised to choose your footwear wisely and avoid these forms if you want to keep back pain at bay.

Smoking

Cigarettes are dangerous not just for your lungs and heart, but also for your back. It has been observed that the incidence of backache in higher in smokers. This can be attributed to the nicotine present in cigarettes that restricts the blood flow to the vertebrae and disks thus depriving them of the essential nutrients. This can cause these structures to age prematurely and prone to breakage.
Now that you have learned the different causes that can lead to back pain, you can surely take steps to avoid most of them. In the next chapter, we will learn some simple exercises you can perform to strengthen your back muscles and avoid backache.

Chapter 2: Simple exercises to prevent the causes of back pain

Exercises offer a great way to relieve back pain. The exercises mentioned beneath are aimed at improving the back support and making the muscles in the region stronger. Let us have a look at them one by one.

Though these exercises involve the neck and shoulder regions as well, they are aimed at strengthening your core and the entire body balance to ensure less pressure is exerted eventually on your back.

Pelvic Bridging

- Lie down on a flat and hard surface on your back. Bend your knees only as much as you feel comfortable.

- Let the arms rest flat on the sides. Slowly, lift your pelvis upward and hold for 4 to 5 seconds and then, relax and come down to the initial position.

- While lifting upwards, breathe in deeply and while coming down breathe out slowly. Repeat 10 to 15 times.

Spine Extension Exercise

- Lie down on your stomach and prop the upper body up on the elbows. Allow the pelvis to sag down while extending the neck backward.

- Then, breathe in as you maintain the position. Exhale slowly and come back to the initial position. Remember not to lift hips.

Pelvic Rolling

- Lie down on a hard surface on your back. Then, bend your knees comfortably and close them together.

- Roll the knees to one side followed by your pelvis and hold for 5 seconds. Then, bring it to initial position. Repeat the same on the other side.

- Make sure your head rotates on the opposite side of the movement of pelvis and knees. Also, your chin should be tucked in and the upper body relaxed.

Knee To Chest

- Lie down on a flat and hard surface on your back. Then, bring one knee closer to the chest. Grasp the lower part of your thigh and bend only until you feel comfortable.

- Hold this position for about 5 seconds and release. Repeat on another leg. Perform this exercise 10 times with each leg.

- Remember that you must lower the legs completely while relaxing.

Coccyx Exercise

- Squeeze together the buttocks to bring them close to each other. Then, hold the position for 5 seconds.

- Repeat 10 times.

Prone Leg Raise

- Lie down on your stomach. Keep both the hands under your forehead such that the head rests on your forearms.

- Then, lift one leg off the ground and extend it as much as you can without feeling any discomfort.

- Make sure your pelvis is not lifted or tilted while doing so. Hold the position for 4 to 5 seconds and then, relax. Repeat the same with the other leg.

- Perform this exercise 10 times with each leg.

Elbow Planks

- Lie on your stomach and lift the body on your elbow. Keep the shoulders at the top of the elbows.

- Then, keeping the knees straight, point the toes downward. Squeeze the buttocks and slowly, breathe in. Maintain this position for about 10 to 15 seconds and relax.

Side Planks

- Lie down on one side with one foot resting on the other. Your elbow should be under the shoulder.

- Now, lift the hips up so that they form a straight line between your groin, and legs through the middle of your neck. Hold this position for 15 to 20 seconds

- Repeat 10 times

Reverse Planks

- Lie on the back keeping the palms under your shoulder. Your heels should be touching the ground.

- Now, lift the body up by pressing your palms and heels against the ground. At the same time, drive the hips up towards the ceiling such that the body takes a linear shape from the ankles to shoulders.

- Hold this position for a few seconds or till you feel comfortable.

- Repeat 10 times.

Resistance Exercises

- Clasp your fingers and place them on your forehead. Try to push the forehead in the front without moving your head or hand.

- Repeat the same by keeping your hand at the back of the head.

- Then, keep the palm of the left hand at the left side of the head and exert pressure on the head with the hand without moving both. Repeat on the other side.

- While applying pressure, hold the position for about 5 seconds. Then, relax for 2 seconds.

- Repeat the activity 10 times on each side.

Wall Push Ups

- Hold your palms against the wall at the shoulder level. Keep them about shoulder-width apart.

- Now, try to push the wall by bending the elbow. Hold the position for 5 to 10 seconds.

- Repeat 10 times.

Shoulder Shrugs

- Slowly bring the shoulders upwards and hold the position for 5 to 10 seconds.

- Repeat the same 10 times.

Practice these exercises regularly to relieve back pain naturally. However, do not go overboard with any of them. The idea is to begin slowly and develop over a period of time.

Stop the activities if you feel even the slightest discomfort. Practice only till you feel comfortable. Over a few days or weeks, you will be able to follow these exercises with better ease and obtain considerable relief from backache.

Chapter 3: How to improve your posture to avoid back pain

While watching television or working in the office, you slouch in your chair or recliner as you burry yourself in the show or try to hurriedly finish the report.

No big deal, right?

Wrong!

It is these habits that have been responsible for causing neck pain. Not paying proper attention to your posture while sitting, sleeping or walking are the major causes of a chronic backache. And hence, the most effective way to relieve this symptom begins with correcting your posture.

In this chapter, we will have a look at the right posture you should adopt to keep your back muscles at ease and prevent a backache.

How does a poor posture provoke back pain?

You may not feel the ill-effects of your wrong posture after sitting for a few hours. However, over time, it can cause immense pressure on your spine leading to anatomical changes in your back.

This, in turn, can trigger back pain by causing constriction of the nerves and blood vessels in the back as well as stiffening of the muscles. Additionally, the strain from poor posture can also cause damage to the discs, and joints resulting in chronic back pain.

Back pain caused due to a poor posture has the following characteristic features:

- It worsens at specific times of the day

- The pain starts in the neck and moves down towards the upper and lower back

- Pain subsides after changing to a comfortable position while standing or sitting

- The pain has a history of sudden onset beginning at a specific event or incident, which coincides with a new job, a new car or a new office chair.

Let us continue with learning the right posture while sitting to avoid strain and the resulting backache.

How to maintain a good posture while sitting?

- When sitting on the chair at a desk, keep your arms flexed at an angle of about 75 to 90 degrees at the elbows. Adjust the chair to maintain this angle.

- Make sure your back is aligned with the back of the chair.

- Avoid leaning forward and slouching even when you are tired from sitting in the chair for a longer duration. Instead, get up and walk about for a few minutes to release the strain and avoid muscle stiffness.

- Sit on the chair with your shoulders straight.

- Keep both the feet touched to the floor. The feet should rest on the floor flat. If you have a problem with your feet reaching the floor, add a footrest to the chair to rest your feet on.

- Your knees should be slightly higher or even with the hips while sitting on the chair.

- Avoid sitting in one place for too long.

How to maintain a good posture while standing?

- Stand with the body weight falling on the balls of the feet, and not on the heels.

- Let your arms hang down naturally along the sides of the body.

- Keep your feet apart slightly at about a shoulder-width distance.

- Tuck the chin in slightly to keep the head level

- Do not lock the knees.

- Stand tall and straight keeping your shoulders upright.

- Be sure your head is squarely held on the top of the spine, and not pushed forward.

- If you have to stand for prolonged hours, shift the weight from one foot to another, or try to rock from the heels to toes.

How to maintain a good posture while walking?

- Keep the shoulders aligned with the rest of the body.

- Avoid pushing your head forward while walking.

- Keep your head up and eyes looking straight in the front.

How to maintain a good posture while driving?

- Sit straight with your back firmly in contact with the back of the seat.

- Adjust the seat to maintain an appropriate distance between you and the steering wheel and pedals to avoid having to lean forward.

- Make sure the headrest supports the middle part of the head and holds it upright. Tilt it forward, if needed, to ensure the head-to-headrest distance is less than four inches.

How to maintain a good posture while lifting and carrying?

- Use the muscles of the stomach and legs for lifting, and not the lower back muscles.

- Make sure you bend at the knees, and not the waist.

- While carrying a large or heavy object, hold it close to your chest.

- If required, use a supportive belt to maintain a good posture while lifting.

- While carrying a purse or backpack, make sure it is as light as possible. If it is heavy, balance the weight on both the sides as much as possible, or switch the sides from time to time.

- When carrying an object with one arm, try to switch the arms frequently to avoid excess strain on one.

- While carrying a backpack, do not lean forward or bend the shoulders. In case, the weight is causing strain, use a rolling backpack with wheels.

How to maintain a good posture while sleeping?

- A relatively firm mattress is the best for ensuring proper back support, though individual preferences are equally important. Make a note of your sleeping position and relate it to the occurrence of back pain to arrive at the most comfortable position for you while sleeping.

- Usually, sleeping on the sides or back is more comfortable and less strenuous for the back than sleeping on the stomach.

- Provide proper support to the back using a pillow.

- Make sure the pillow offers proper alignment for your head and shoulders.

- You may put a rolled-up towel under your neck and a pillow under your knees for an improved support for your spine.

- When sleeping on the sides, place a relatively flat pillow between your legs to keep the spine straight and aligned.

It is important to note that a bad posture can tense the muscles and pull the entire body out of alignment. Hence, it is very important to maintain the right posture to avoid excess strain on the muscles and avoid back pain.

Chapter 4: The basic yoga poses for relieving back pain naturally

Do you remember what did you learn in your first standard when you had just started going to school? Did your teachers teach you the tales of Shakespeare or how to calculate the percentage? No! You began with learning the alphabets and numbers and then, gradually took steps to imbibe more knowledge to be what you are today! Similarly, when you are just beginning tour journey to relieve your back pain with a long-lasting relief, wouldn't it be wise to begin with the basics? Yes, of course! Here are a few basic yoga asanas especially meant for the beginners that will help you start your journey towards relieving back pain and improving your health and fitness with better ease and more confidence.

Balasana

- Kneel down with the top of your feet and the knees on the floor. Keep your feet touching each other.

- Now, keep your knees apart, and then, rest your chest and belly between legs and then, gently place your head on the floor.

- Stretch out the arms in the front. Use a pillow to rest on if your head can not reach the floor.

- This basic move forms a resting pose in which you can stay for a few minutes between 2 poses.

Utkatasana

- Stand straight with your feet touching. You can keep them a few inches apart if you're stiff.

- Then, bend your knees as if you are sitting on a chair and raise your arms alongside your ears.

- Feel free to relax out of the pose. Do this 5 times.

- This one is a symmetrical pose, which means it will allow both sides of your body to move in and out at the same time. It strengthens the legs and heats you up.

Adho Mukha Svanasana

- Bend forward at the waist with your feet a few inches apart.

- Then, press your palms into the ground. At this moment, your hands should be stretched apart and the shoulders, arms, and back should be in a straight, diagonal line.

- Keep the hands at the front and the toes facing backward.

- Keep in the pose for 15 seconds and then release.

- Do this 5 times to begin with and then, increase gradually.

- Bending your knees slightly is an accepted modification especially for those with tight hamstrings

Vrksasana

- Stand on one leg. Then, bring the foot near the ankle or shin depending on your flexibility.

- Put your hands against the wall for balance or stand with your back resting against a wall.

- Once you are able to achieve a balance, lift your arms up into the air.

- Do this 5 times every day.

Salabhasana

- Lie down on your belly and inhale. Raise your body while inhaling. Keep your palms facing the floor.

- Focus on extending the head up and keeping your neck long.

- Clasp your hands firmly behind your back while lifting your limbs so as to create a deeper opening for the shoulders and chest.

- Stay in the pose for 5 seconds and then release. Do this 5 times every day.

Shavasana

- Lie down flat on your back. Close the eyes and try to relax your body. Keep your legs hip-width apart and rest your arms at an angle of 45-degrees to the torso. The palms should be facing up.

- Allow the limbs to relax completely. Place a folded blanket below the knees if you want more space for your back.

Setu Bandha Sarvangasana

- Lie down flat on the floor with your knees bent and feet flat touching the floor.

- The knees should be pointing up to the ceiling.

- Keep your hands alongside your body.

- Then, with your feet on the ground, press into your hands and move the hips away from the floor. You can hold your mat with your hands.

- It gives a leverage to turn the arms so that your palms are facing up.

- Do this 5 times and then, increase gradually.

Tadasana

- Stand straight with your feet close to each other. Make sure your big toes are touching each other and keep your eyes closed.

- Separate your feet slightly if you feel stiff. Then, rest your arms at your sides.

- If you find standing to be a challenge, then lie down on your back and press up the soles of your feet against a wall.

- This way; you'll feel as if you're standing on the floor. Do this 2 to 3 times.

Viparita Karani

- Lie down on your back and slowly walk the legs up over a wall.

- Keep your legs straight and make sure your back meets the wall. You can place a pillow under your back for added support.

- You may experience tingling in your legs especially when you're new to this position.

- Ride your legs down the wall and pull your knees to the chest to get rid of this sensation. You can also stretch your feet up the wall.

- Do this 5 times every day.

Virabhadrasana II

- Stand with your feet wide apart. Turn your right leg outward in 90 degrees and angle in your left toes slightly.

- Then, take out your arms to the side till they level with the floor.

- Bend your right knee making it stack on the top of your ankle. Make an imaginary square with your right knee and hold the pose. If it's too difficult to hold for long, come in and out of the position with each breath.

- Repeat for the opposite side. Do this 3 to 4 times.

Though these poses are meant for the beginners, it doesn't mean they are anyway less in providing a remarkable relief from back pain. You can continue practicing these poses every day for about 20 minutes to stay fit and healthy and to prevent diseases.

Chapter 5: Alternative treatments for long-term relief from back pain

Alternative therapies such as acupressure, Ayurveda, and massage can help relieve back pain by creating a deep relaxation of the muscles and correcting the deeply rooted imbalances in the body. These therapies are aimed at restoring harmony and functional integrity in the body.

In this chapter, we will have a look at the alternative therapies, and some lifestyle changes recommended to improve general health and prevent chronic disorders such as back pain.

Massage therapies

Massage of the back using medicated oils by inducing long, vigorous strokes can revitalize the tissues and cells in the bones, and muscles. A massage can also soothe the nerves and strengthen the bones. It can create a sense of tranquility in the mind, delay the process of aging and reduce the risk of complications associated with chronic back pain.

Some more benefits of massage therapies include:

- Eases muscular aches and pains while promoting muscle relaxation

- Improves blood circulation and lymphatic drainage

- Eliminates toxins from the body

- Stimulates the immune power and strengthens the resistance to infections

- Alleviates potential adverse effects of stress

Massage therapy can be performed using warm medicated, herbal oils. The massage is focused on calming the nerves and muscles and relieving stiffness. A complete body massage is also recommended to improve the ability of nutrients to reach all the cells and remove stagnant waste.

A massage of the back using a concoction of warm herbal oils can nourish and revitalize the tissues. This treatment produces a deep healing effect by bringing harmony into the body, mind, and spirit, naturally.

Acupressure

Acupressure is a unique alternative treatment for healing back pain without the risk of any side effects. The all you need to do is apply firm pressure on some specific points and you will get remarkable relief from the symptoms.

The acupressure therapy can not only provide instant relief from back pain, but also prevent it from coming up again and again.

However, you must learn the proper technique of applying pressure on the acupressure points for relieving back pain. Some of the most effective acupressure points for reducing back pain are as follows:

Stomach Point

Stomach point is helpful for reducing pain in the lower back. The point is situated 2 fingers below the belly button. The stomach point is also called the Sea of Energy point.

Apply firm pressure on the stomach point for a few seconds every day. It will help to reduce weakness of the lower back and strengthen the abdominal muscles. This will lessen the strain or pressure on the muscles of the back and prevent backache.

Lower Back Points

Applying pressure on the lower back points can give instant relief from the lower back pain and sciatica. Acupressure points in the lower back are located near the spine at the waist level. These points are also called the Sea of Vitality. The point is situated between the second and third lumbar vertebrae.

Applying firm pressure on this point will release the stiffness of the muscles in the lower back significantly.

Hipbone Points

Hipbone points for back pain are impactful for reducing pelvic tension and hip pain. These acupressure points are situated near the hipbone at the middle part of the top of the hip bone and the base of the buttock. Applying gentle pressure on this point will relieve lower back pain, pelvic stress, and sciatica.

Eat right to keep the spine strong

Healthy eating habits form an important aspect of keeping your spine strong. Eat foods rich in calcium and vitamin D such as milk, yogurt, fatty fish, leafy vegetables, and egg. This will nourish the body and prevent the deficiency of essential vitamins, and minerals that are responsible for triggering back pain.

Reduce mental stress

You may not realize this, but stress can be a major factor responsible for stiffness of the muscles in the back resulting in chronic pain. By reducing mental stress, you can obtain significant relief from back pain. Some of the most effective stress-busting methods include yoga, meditation, and deep breathing exercises.

Quit smoking

Smoking is injurious not just for your lungs but also for your back. Research studies suggest that nicotine in cigarettes can narrow the blood vessels in the spinal column. This can result in a reduced supply of essential nutrients and oxygen to the vertebra, spine, and the muscles in the back causing back pain.

Watch your pounds

Being obese or overweight can contribute to a bad posture and lead to back pain. Keep in mind that each extra pound in your body, especially around the midsection, causes its center of gravity to shift backward thus forcing you to adopt a faulty posture to maintain balance. Hence, if you are obese, consider reducing weight by adopting healthy eating habits, and exercising regularly.

These strategies seem to be too simple. But, the benefits can be huge. Make sure you follow the strategies given here to keep back pain at bay.

Conclusion

Keeping your back happy and healthy can be easy if you make some simple changes in your lifestyle. I strongly believe that your own lifestyle habits are responsible for your health. If you follow healthy ways of living your life with regular exercises, and eating nutritious foods, you can easily avoid back pain.

Maintaining the right posture while sitting, standing, walking, sleeping, etc. can help relieve back pain to a great extent. Performing the exercises that relieve back pain on a regular basis can also keep the back muscles free of stiffness and enable pain-less movements.

The management of back pain can be coupled with the yoga asanas and the alternative treatments such as massage therapies and acupressure for better and faster results.

Adopting the right lifestyle and following the tips mentioned in this book can provide an all-encompassing treatment for chronic back pain!

So, why wait? Begin with the simple yoga poses, and start exercising regularly to get going on the path of healthier and happier back!

Good luck!

Thank you again for downloading this book!

I hope this book was able to help you to get relief from back pain.

Finally, if you enjoyed this book, then I'd like to ask you for a favor, would you be kind enough to leave a review for this book on Amazon? It'd be greatly appreciated!

Thank you and good luck!